My Air Fryer Cookbook
A Handful of Quick, Delicious Recipes for Your Air Fryer Meals

Eva Sheppard

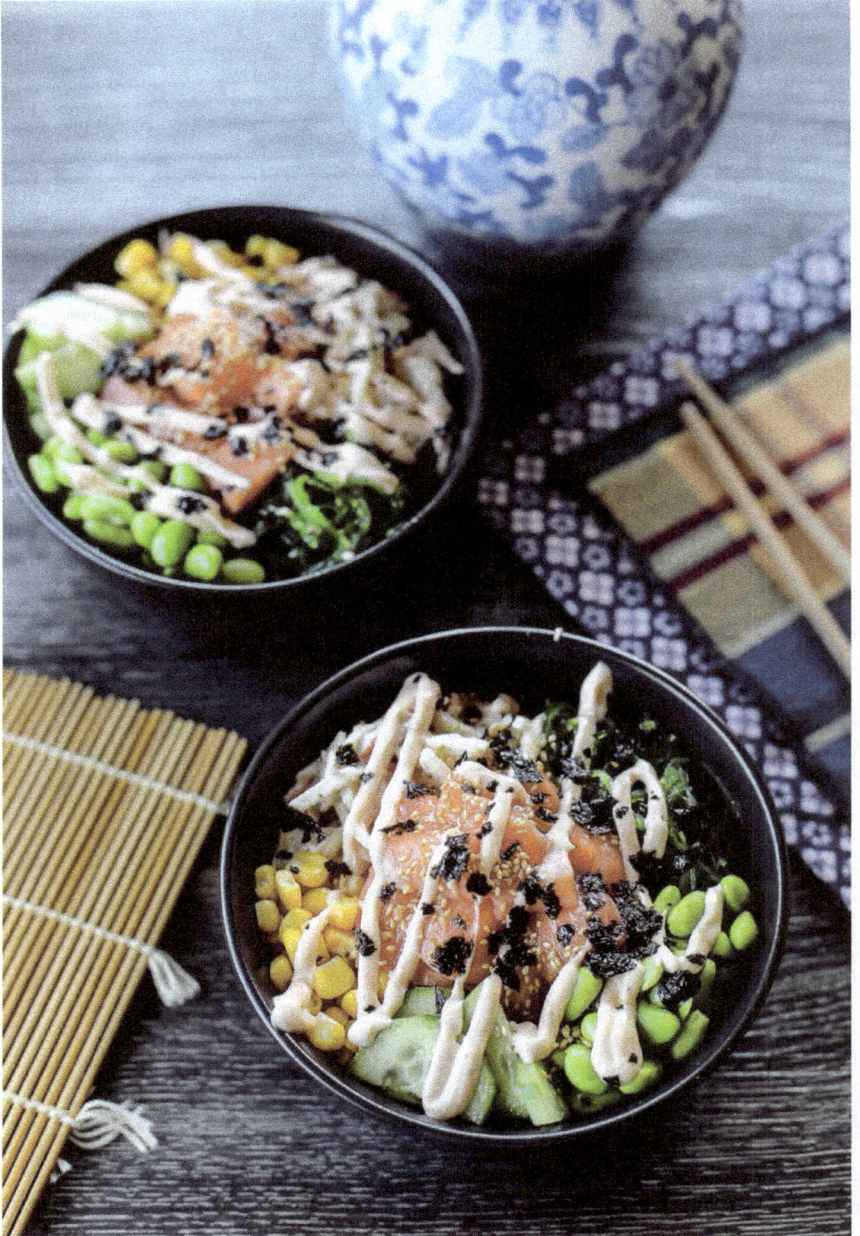

not engaging in the rendering of legal, financial, medical or professional advice. The content within this book has been derived from various sources. Please consult a licensed professional before attempting any techniques outlined in this book.

By reading this document, the reader agrees that under no circumstances is the author responsible for any losses, direct or indirect, which are incurred as a result of the use of information contained within this document, including, but not limited to, — errors, omissions, or inaccuracies.

TABLE OF CONTENT

6

Balsamic Artichokes Recipe

Preparation Time: 17 Minutes

Servings: 4

Ingredients:

- 4 big artichokes; trimmed
- 2 tbsp. lemon juice
- 2 tsp. balsamic vinegar
- 1 tsp. oregano; dried
- 1/4 cup extra virgin olive oil
- 2 garlic cloves; minced
- Salt and black pepper to the taste

Directions:

1. Season artichokes with salt and pepper, rub them with half of the oil and half of the lemon juice, put them in your air fryer and cook at 360 °F, for 7 minutes

2. Meanwhile; in a bowl, mix the rest of the lemon juice with vinegar, the remaining oil, salt, pepper, garlic and oregano and stir very well

3. Arrange artichokes on a platter, drizzle the balsamic vinaigrette over them and serve.

Nutrition Values: Calories: 200; Fat: 3; Fiber: 6; Carbs: 12; Protein: 4

Beets and Arugula Salad time Recipe

Preparation Time: 20 Minutes

Servings: 4

Ingredients:

- 1 ½ lbs. beets; peeled and quartered
- 2 tbsp. brown sugar
- 2 scallions; chopped
- 2 tsp. mustard
- A drizzle of olive oil
- 2 tsp. orange zest; grated
- 2 tbsp. cider vinegar
- 1/2 cup orange juice
- 2 cups arugula

Directions:

1. Rub beets with the oil and orange juice, place them in your air fryer and cook at 350 °F, for 10 minutes

2. Transfer beet quarters to a bowl, add scallions, arugula and orange zest and toss

3. In a separate bowl, mix sugar with mustard and vinegar, whisk well, add to salad, toss and serve.

Nutrition Values: Calories: 121; Fat: 2; Fiber: 3; Carbs: 11; Protein: 4

Sesame Mustard Greens Recipe

Preparation Time: 21 Minutes

Servings: 4

Ingredients:

- 2 garlic cloves; minced
- 3 tbsp. veggie stock
- 1/4 tsp. dark sesame oil
- 1 lb. mustard greens; torn
- 1 tbsp. olive oil
- 1/2 cup yellow onion; sliced
- Salt and black pepper to the taste

Directions:

1. Heat up a pan that fits your air fryer with the oil over medium heat, add onions; stir and brown them for 5 minutes.

2. Add garlic, stock, greens, salt and pepper; stir, introduce in your air fryer and cook at

350 °F, for 6 minutes. Add sesame oil, toss to coat, divide among plates and serve

Nutrition Values: Calories: 120; Fat: 3; Fiber: 1; Carbs: 3; Protein: 7

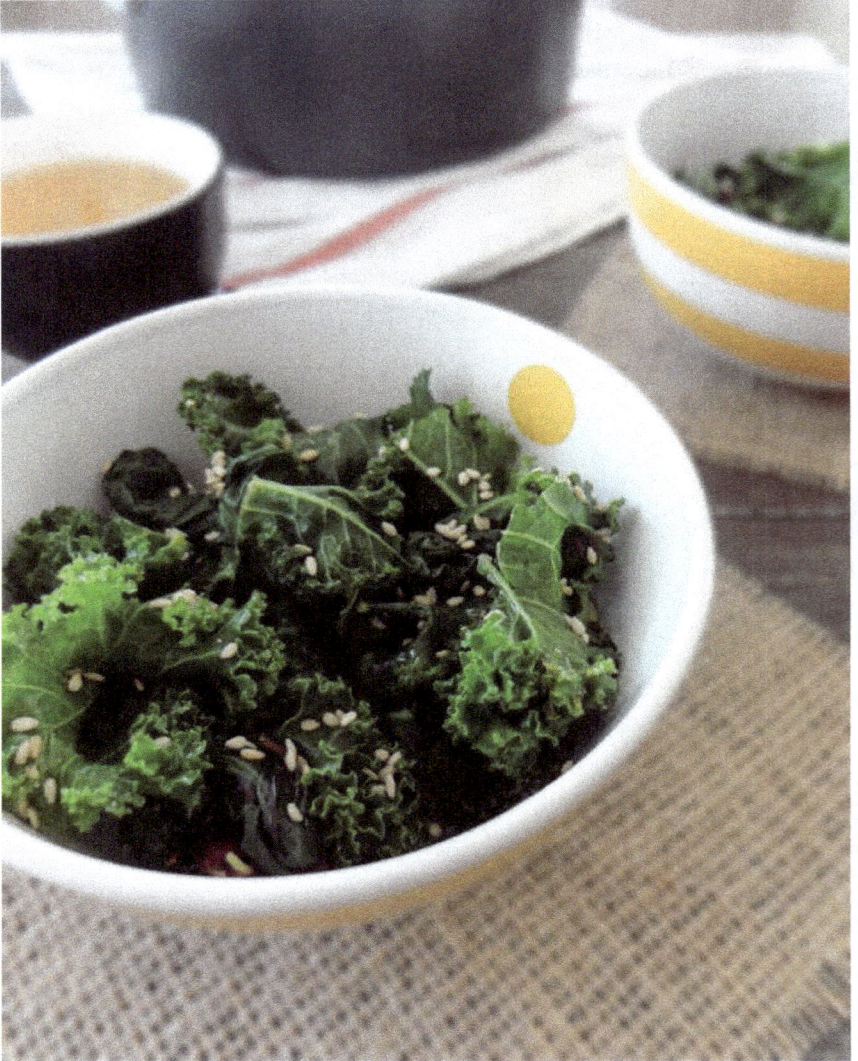

Garlic Tomatoes Recipe

Preparation Time: 25 Minutes

Servings: 4

Ingredients:

- 4 garlic cloves; crushed

- 1 lb. mixed cherry tomatoes

- 3 thyme springs; chopped.

- 1/4 cup olive oil

- Salt and black pepper to the taste

Directions:

1. In a bowl; mix tomatoes with salt, black pepper, garlic, olive oil and thyme, toss to coat, introduce in your air fryer and cook at 360 °F, for 15 minutes. Divide tomatoes mix on plates and serve

Nutrition Values: Calories: 100; Fat: 0; Fiber: 1; Carbs: 1; Protein: 6

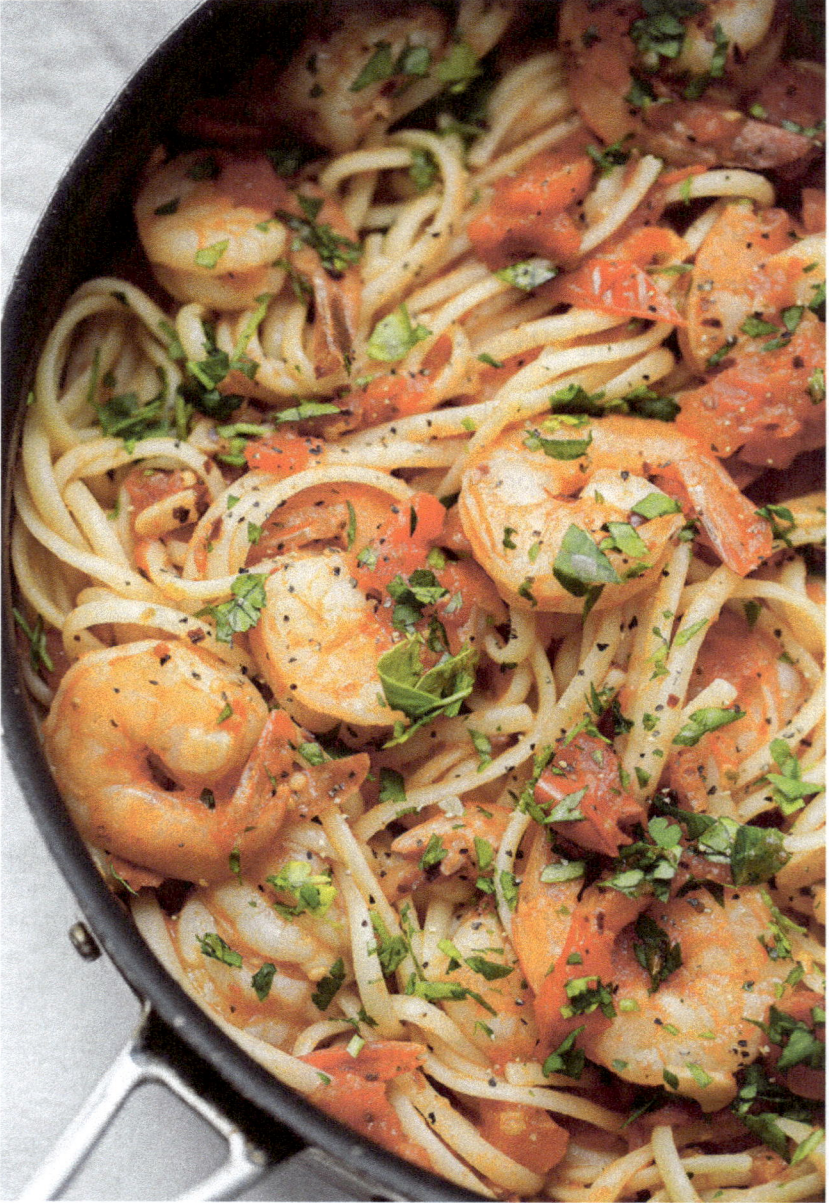

Broccoli and Tomatoes Fried Stew Recipe

Preparation Time: 30 Minutes

Servings: 4

Ingredients:

- 28 oz. canned tomatoes; pureed
- 1 broccoli head; florets separated
- 2 tsp. coriander seeds
- 1 tbsp. olive oil
- 1 yellow onion; chopped
- A pinch of red pepper; crushed
- 1 small ginger piece; chopped
- 1 garlic clove; minced
- Salt and black pepper to the taste

Directions:

1. Heat up a pan that fits your air fryer with the oil over medium heat, add onions, salt, pepper and red pepper; stir and cook for 7 minutes

2. Add ginger, garlic, coriander seeds, tomatoes and broccoli; stir, introduce in your air fryer and cook at 360 °F, for 12 minutes. Divide into bowls and serve.

Nutrition Values: Calories: 150; Fat: 4; Fiber: 2; Carbs: 7; Protein: 12

Cheesy Artichokes Recipe

Preparation Time: 16 Minutes

Servings: 6

Ingredients:

- 14 oz. canned artichoke hearts
- 8 oz. cream cheese
- 8 oz. mozzarella; shredded
- 1/2 cup sour cream
- 3 garlic cloves; minced
- 16 oz. parmesan cheese; grated
- 10 oz. spinach
- 1/2 cup chicken stock
- 1/2 cup mayonnaise
- 1 tsp. onion powder

Directions:

1. In a pan that fits your air fryer, mix artichokes with stock, garlic, spinach, cream cheese, sour cream, onion powder and mayo, toss, introduce in your air fryer and cook at 350 °F, for 6 minutes

2. Add mozzarella and parmesan; stir well and serve.

Nutrition Values: Calories: 261; Fat: 12; Fiber: 2; Carbs: 12; Protein: 15

Stuffed Eggplants Recipe

Preparation Time: 40 Minutes

Servings: 4

Ingredients:

- 4 small eggplants; halved lengthwise
- 1/2 cup cauliflower; chopped.
- 1 tsp. oregano; chopped
- 1/2 cup parsley; chopped
- Salt and black pepper to the taste
- 10 tbsp. olive oil
- 2 ½ lbs. tomatoes; cut into halves and grated
- 1 green bell pepper; chopped.
- 1 yellow onion; chopped
- 1 tbsp. garlic; minced
- 3 oz. feta cheese; crumbled

Directions:

1. Season eggplants with salt, pepper and 4 tbsp. oil, toss, put them in your air fryer and cook at 350 °F, for 16 minutes.

2. Meanwhile; heat up a pan with 3 tbsp. oil over medium high heat, add onion; stir and cook for 5 minutes.

3. Add bell pepper, garlic and cauliflower; stir, cook for 5 minutes; take off heat, add parsley, tomato, salt, pepper, oregano and cheese and whisk everything

4. Stuff eggplants with the veggie mix, drizzle the rest of the oil over them, put them in your air fryer and cook at 350 °F, for 6 minutes more. Divide among plates and serve right away

Nutrition Values: Calories: 240; Fat: 4, fiber, 2; Carbs: 19; Protein: 2

Fried Asparagus Recipe

Preparation Time: 25 Minutes

Servings: 4

Ingredients:

- 2 lbs. fresh asparagus; trimmed
- 1/2 tsp. oregano; dried
- 1/4 tsp. red pepper flakes
- 1/4 cup olive oil
- Salt and black pepper to the taste
- 1 tsp. lemon zest
- 4 oz. feta cheese; crumbled
- 4 garlic cloves; minced
- 2 tbsp. parsley; finely chopped.
- Juice from 1 lemon

Directions:

1. In a bowl; mix oil with lemon zest, garlic, pepper flakes and oregano and whisk.

2. Add asparagus, cheese, salt and pepper, toss, transfer to your air fryer's basket and cook at 350 °F, for 8 minutes.

3. Divide asparagus on plates, drizzle lemon juice and sprinkle parsley on top and serve

Nutrition Values: Calories: 162; Fat: 13; Fiber: 5; Carbs: 12; Protein: 8

Collard Greens Mix Recipe

Preparation Time: 20 Minutes

Servings: 4

Ingredients:

- 1 bunch collard greens; trimmed
- 2 tbsp. olive oil
- 2 tbsp. tomato puree
- 1 tbsp. balsamic vinegar
- 1 tsp. sugar
- 1 yellow onion; chopped
- 3 garlic cloves; minced
- Salt and black pepper to the taste

Directions:

1. In a dish that fits your air fryer, mix oil, garlic, vinegar, onion and tomato puree and whisk

2. Add collard greens, salt, pepper and sugar, toss, introduce in your air fryer and cook at

320 °F, for 10 minutes. Divide collard greens mix on plates and serve

Nutrition Values: Calories: 121; Fat: 3; Fiber: 3; Carbs: 7; Protein: 3

Spanish Greens Recipe

Preparation Time: 18 Minutes

Servings: 4

Ingredients:

- 1 apple; cored and chopped.
- 1 yellow onion; sliced
- 1/4 cup pine nuts; toasted
- 1/4 cup balsamic vinegar
- 3 tbsp. olive oil
- 1/4 cup raisins
- 6 garlic cloves; chopped
- 5 cups mixed spinach and chard
- Salt and black pepper to the taste
- A pinch of nutmeg

Directions:

1. Heat up a pan that fits your air fryer with the oil over medium high heat, add onion; stir and cook for 3 minutes

2. Add apple, garlic, raisins, vinegar, mixed spinach and chard, nutmeg, salt and pepper; stir, introduce in preheated air fryer and cook at 350 °F, for 5 minutes

3. Divide among plates, sprinkle pine nuts on top and serve.

Nutrition Values: Calories: 120; Fat: 1; Fiber: 2; Carbs: 3; Protein: 6

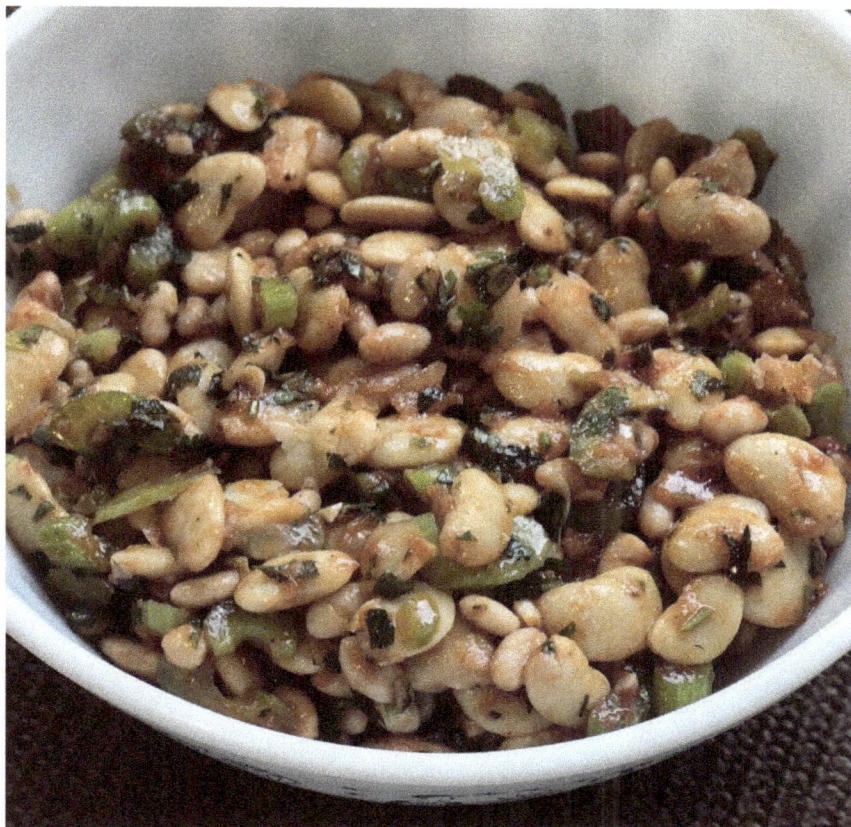

Stuffed Tomatoes Recipe

Preparation Time: 25 Minutes

Servings: 4

Ingredients:

- 4 tomatoes; tops cut off and pulp scooped and chopped.
- 1 yellow onion; chopped.
- 1 tbsp. butter
- 2 tbsp. celery; chopped
- 1/2 cup mushrooms; chopped.
- 1 tbsp. bread crumbs
- 1 cup cottage cheese
- Salt and black pepper to the taste
- 1/4 tsp. caraway seeds
- 1 tbsp. parsley; chopped

Directions:

1. Heat up a pan with the butter over medium heat, melt it, add onion and celery; stir and cook for 3 minutes.

2. Add tomato pulp and mushrooms; stir and cook for 1 minute more

3. Add salt, pepper, crumbled bread, cheese, caraway seeds and parsley; stir, cook for 4 minutes more and take off heat.

4. Stuff tomatoes with this mix, place them in your air fryer and cook at 350 °F, for 8 minutes. Divide stuffed tomatoes on plates and serve

Nutrition Values: Calories: 143; Fat: 4; Fiber: 6; Carbs: 4; Protein: 4

Zucchini Mix Recipe

Preparation Time: 24 Minutes

Servings: 6

Ingredients:

- 6 zucchinis; halved and then sliced

- 3 garlic cloves; minced

- 2 oz. parmesan; grated

- 3/4 cup heavy cream

- Salt and black pepper to the taste

- 1 tbsp. butter

- 1 tsp. oregano; dried

- 1/2 cup yellow onion; chopped

Directions:

1. Heat up a pan that fits your air fryer with the butter over medium high heat, add onion; stir and cook for 4 minutes

2. Add garlic, zucchinis, oregano, salt, pepper and heavy cream, toss, introduce in your air fryer and cook at 350 °F, for 10 minutes.

Add parmesan; stir, divide among plates and serve.

Nutrition Values: Calories: 160; Fat: 4; Fiber: 2; Carbs: 8; Protein: 8

Broccoli Hash Recipe

Preparation Time: 38 Minutes

Servings: 2

Ingredients:

- 10 oz. mushrooms; halved
- 1 broccoli head; florets separated
- 1 garlic clove; minced
- 1 tbsp. balsamic vinegar
- 1 avocado; peeled and pitted
- A pinch of red pepper flakes
- 1 yellow onion; chopped.
- 1 tbsp. olive oil
- Salt and black pepper
- 1 tsp. basil; dried

Directions:

1. In a bowl; mix mushrooms with broccoli, onion, garlic and avocado.

2. In another bowl, mix vinegar, oil, salt, pepper and basil and whisk well

3. Pour this over veggies, toss to coat, leave aside for 30 minutes; transfer to your air fryer's basket and cook at 350 °F, for 8 minutes; Divide among plates and serve with pepper flakes on top

Nutrition Values: Calories: 182; Fat: 3; Fiber: 3; Carbs: 5; Protein: 8

Grilled Lamb with Herbed Salt

Servings: 8

Cooking Time: 1 hour 20 minutes

Ingredients:

- 4 pounds boneless leg of lamb, cut into 2-inch chunks
- 2 ½ tablespoons herb salt
- 2 tablespoons olive oil

Directions:

1. Preheat the air fryer at 3900F.

2. Place the grill pan accessory in the air fryer.

3. Season the meat with the herb salt and brush with olive oil.

4. Grill the meat for 20 minutes per batch.

5. Make sure to flip the meat every 10 minutes for even cooking.

Nutrition Values:

Calories: 347; Carbs: 0g; Protein: 46.6g; Fat: 17.8g

Delicious Dry Rubbed Flank Steak

Servings: 3

Cooking Time: 45 minutes

Ingredients:

- 2 tablespoons sugar
- 1 tablespoon chili powder
- 1 tablespoon paprika
- 2 teaspoons salt
- 2 teaspoons black pepper
- 1 teaspoon garlic powder
- 1 teaspoon mustard powder
- ½ teaspoon coriander
- ½ teaspoon ground cumin
- 1 ½ pounds flank steak

Directions:

1. Preheat the air fryer at 3900F.

2. Place the grill pan accessory in the air fryer.

3. In a small bowl, combine all the spices and rub all over the flank steak.

4. Place on the grill and cook for 15 minutes per batch.

5. Make sure to flip the meat every 8 minutes for even grilling.

Nutrition Values:

Calories: 330; Carbs: 10.2g; Protein:50 g; Fat:12.1 g

Grilled Leg of Lamb with Mint Yogurt

Servings: 6

Cooking Time: 1 hour

Ingredients:

- 1 cup rosemary leaves
- ¾ cup peeled garlic cloves, crushed
- 2 tablespoons olive oil
- 3 pounds lamb shanks, boned removed and sliced into 2-inch chunks
- 1 tablespoon lemon zest
- Salt and pepper to taste
- 2 cups Greek yogurt
- 1 cup fresh mint, chopped
- 1 tablespoon lemon juice

Directions:

1. Place in the Ziploc bag the rosemary leaves, garlic cloves, olive oil, lamb shanks, and

lemon zest. Season with salt and pepper to taste.

2. Allow to marinate for 30 minutes in the fridge.
3. Preheat the air fryer at 3900F.
4. Place the grill pan accessory in the air fryer.
5. Place the lamb shanks and garlic on the grill pan and cook for 20 minutes per batch.
6. Flip the meat every 10 minutes.
7. Meanwhile, mix together the Greek yogurt, fresh mint, and lemon juice. Season with salt and pepper to taste.
8. Serve the lamb shanks with the mint yogurt

Nutrition Values:

Calories: 443; Carbs: 9.6g; Protein: 63.9g; Fat: 16.5g

Grilled Steak with Beet Salad

Servings: 6

Cooking Time: 45 minutes

Ingredients:

- 1-pound tri-tip, sliced
- 2 tablespoons olive oil
- Salt and pepper to taste
- 1 bunch scallions, chopped
- 1 bunch arugula, torn
- 3 beets, peeled and sliced thinly
- 3 tablespoons balsamic vinegar

Directions:

1. Preheat the air fryer at 3900F.

2. Place the grill pan accessory in the air fryer.

3. Season the tri-tip with salt and pepper. Drizzle with oil.

4. Grill for 15 minutes per batch.

5. Meanwhile, prepare the salad by tossing the rest of the ingredients in a salad bowl.

6. Toss in the grilled tri-trip and drizzle with more balsamic vinegar.

Nutrition Values:

Calories: 221; Carbs: 20.7g; Protein: 17.2g; Fat: 7.7g

Grilled Sweet and Sour Soy Pork Belly

Servings: 4

Cooking Time: 60 minutes

Ingredients:

- 2 pounds pork belly
- ¼ cup lemon juice
- ½ cup soy sauce
- 3 tablespoons brown sugar
- 2 tablespoons hoisin sauce
- Salt and pepper to taste
- 3-star anise
- 1 bay leaf

Directions:

1. Place all ingredients in a Ziploc bag and allow to marinate in the fridge for at least 2 hours.

2. Preheat the air fryer at 3900F.

3. Place the grill pan accessory in the air fryer.

4. Grill the pork for at least 20 minutes per batch.

5. Make sure to flip the pork every 10 minutes.

6. Chop the pork before serving and garnish with green onions.

Nutrition Values:

Calories: 1301; Carbs: 15.5g; Protein:24 g; Fat: 126.4g

Texas Rodeo-Style Beef

Servings: 6

Cooking Time: 1 hour

Ingredients:

- 3 pounds beef steak sliced
- Salt and pepper to taste
- 2 onion, chopped
- ½ cup honey
- ½ cup ketchup
- 1 clove of garlic, minced
- 1 tablespoon chili powder
- ½ teaspoon dry mustard

Directions:

1. Place all ingredients in a Ziploc bag and allow to marinate in the fridge for at least 2 hours.

2. Preheat the air fryer at 3900F.

3. Place the grill pan accessory in the air fryer.

4. Grill the beef for 15 minutes per batch making sure that you flip it every 8 minutes for even grilling.

5. Meanwhile, pour the marinade on a saucepan and allow to simmer over medium heat until the sauce thickens.

6. Baste the beef with the sauce before serving.

Nutrition Values:

Calories: 542; Carbs: 49g; Protein: 37g; Fat: 22g

Mustard-Marinated Flank Steak

Servings: 3

Cooking Time: 45 minutes

Ingredients:

- 1 ¼ pounds beef flank steak
- ½ teaspoon black pepper
- 1 cup Italian salad dressing
- ½ cup yellow mustard
- Salt to taste

Directions:

1. Place all ingredients in a Ziploc bag and allow to marinate in the fridge for at least 2 hours.

2. Preheat the air fryer at 3900F.

3. Place the grill pan accessory in the air fryer.

4. Grill for 15 minutes per batch making sure to flip the meat halfway through the cooking time.

Nutrition Values:

Calories: 576; Carbs: 3.1g; Protein:35 g; Fat: 47g

Grilled Rum Beef Ribeye Steak

Servings: 4

Cooking Time: 50 minutes

Ingredients:

- 2 pounds bone-in ribeye steak
- 2 tablespoons extra virgin olive oil
- Salt and black pepper to taste
- ½ cup rum

Directions:

1. Place all ingredients in a Ziploc bag and allow to marinate in the fridge for at least 2 hours.

2. Preheat the air fryer at 3900F.

3. Place the grill pan accessory in the air fryer.

4. Grill for 25 minutes per piece.

5. Halfway through the cooking time, flip the meat for even grilling.

Nutrition Values:

Calories: 394; Carbs: 0.1g; Protein: 48.9g; Fat: 21.5g

Yummy and Creamy Squash Mix

Preparation Time: 17 minutes

Servings: 6

Ingredients:

- big butternut squash - 1, roughly cubed
- sour cream - 1 cup
- Salt and black pepper to taste
- Parsley - 1 tablespoon, chopped
- A drizzle of olive oil

Directions:

1. Place the squash in the air fryer, then add the salt and pepper as seasoning. Ensure to rub with oil.

2. Cook at a temperature of 400 o F for about 15 minutes.

3. Then move the squash to a clean bowl before adding the cream and the parsley.

4. Toss well to coat before serving.

Nutrition Values:

calories 200, fat 7, fiber 6, carbs 11, protein 7

Orange Carrots Mix

Preparation Time: 20 minutes

Servings: 4

Ingredients:

- baby carrots - 1½ pounds
- orange zest - 2 teaspoons
- cider vinegar - 2 tablespoons
- orange juice - ½ cup
- A handful of parsley, chopped
- A drizzle of olive oil

Directions:

1. Place the baby carrots in your clean air fryer's basket, followed by addition of the orange zest and oil,. Ensure that you rub the carrots well.

2. Cook at a temperature of 350 o F for 15 minutes.

3. Move the carrots to a clean bowl, before adding the vinegar and orange as well as juice, and parsley.

4. Toss well to coat, serve away, and enjoy your meal!

Nutrition Values:

calories 151, fat 6, fiber 6, carbs 11, protein 5

Tomato Salad Mix

Preparation Time: 10 minutes

Servings: 8

Ingredients:

- red onion - 1, sliced
- feta cheese - 2 ounces, crumbled
- Salt and black pepper to taste
- mixed cherry tomatoes - 1 pint, halved
- pecans - 2 ounces
- olive oil - 2 tablespoons

Directions:

1. Mix the tomatoes with the salt, pepper, onions, and the oil in your air fryer.

2. Cook at a temperature of 400 o F for 5 minutes.

3. Move to a bowl before adding the pecans and the cheese.

4. Toss well to coat and serve away.

Nutrition Values:

calories 151, fat 4, fiber 6, carbs 9, protein 4

Hot Tomato and Green Beans Salad

Preparation Time: 11 minutes

Servings: 4

Ingredients:

- green beans - 1 pound, trimmed and halved
- green onions - 2, chopped
- canned green chilies - 5 ounces, chopped
- jalapeno pepper - 1, chopped
- A drizzle of olive oil
- chili powder - 2 teaspoons
- garlic powder - 1 teaspoon
- Salt and black pepper to taste
- cherry tomatoes - 8, halved

Directions:

1. Put every single ingredient in a pan that fits perfectly into your air fryer, then mix and toss properly.

2. Introduce the pan to the fryer and cook at a temperature of 400 o F for a little above 5 minutes.

3. Cut the mix into different plates and serve while the meal is still hot.

Nutrition Values:

calories 200, fat 4, fiber 7, carbs 12, protein 6

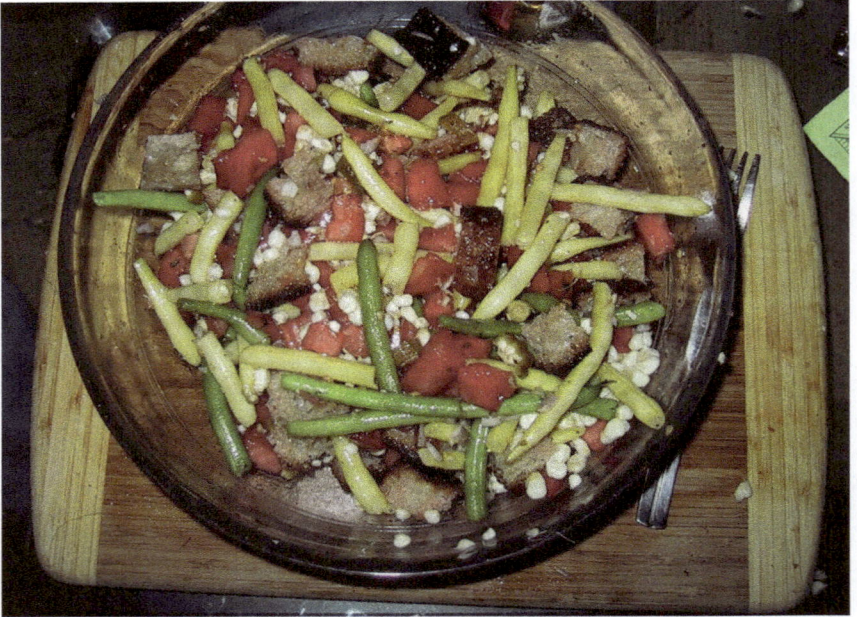

Bell Peppers and Kale Mix

Preparation Time: 20 minutes

Servings: 4

Ingredients:

- red bell peppers - 2, cut into strips
- green bell peppers - 2, cut into strips
- kale leaves - ½ pound
- Salt and black pepper to taste
- yellow onions - 2, roughly chopped
- veggie stock - ¼ cup
- tomato sauce - 2 tablespoons

Directions:

1. Put all of the ingredients in a pan that fits right into your air fryer; then mix well.

2. Transfer the pan to the fryer and cook at a temperature of 360 o F for 15 minutes.

3. Cut into different plates, serve your meal, and enjoy!

Nutrition Values:

calories 161, fat 7, fiber 6, carbs 12, protein 7

Seasoned Garlic Parsnips

Preparation Time: 20 minutes

Servings: 4

Ingredients:

- Parsnips - 1 pound, cut into chunks
- olive oil - 1 tablespoon
- garlic cloves - 6, minced
- balsamic vinegar - 1 tablespoon
- Salt and black pepper to taste

Directions:

1. Put all of the ingredients in a bowl and mix properly.

2. Transfer them to the air fryer and cook at a temperature of 380 o F for 15 minutes.

3. Cut into different plates and serve away.

Nutrition Values:

calories 121, fat 3, fiber 6, carbs 12, protein 6

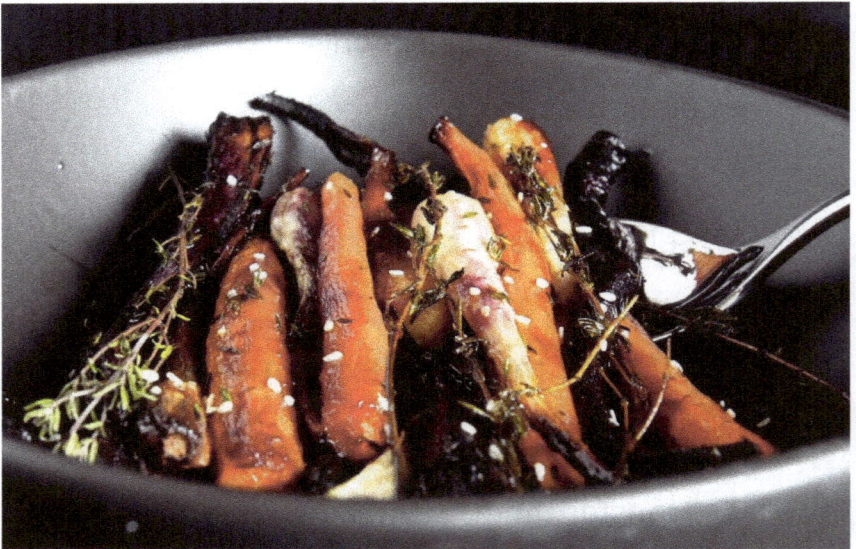

Broccoli and Pomegranate Toppings

Preparation Time: 12 minutes

Servings: 4

Ingredients:

- broccoli head - 1, florets separated
- Salt and black pepper to taste
- Pomegranate - 1, seeds separated
- A drizzle of olive oil

Directions:

1. Mix the broccoli with the salt, pepper, and oil in a bowl; toss well to coat.

2. Introduce the florets to your air fryer and cook at a temperature of 400 o F for a little above 5 minutes.

3. Cut into different plates, sprinkle the pomegranate seeds all over the dish, and serve away.

Nutrition Values:

calories 141, fat 3, fiber 4, carbs 11, protein 4

Hot Bacon Cauliflower

Preparation Time: 12 minutes

Servings: 4

Ingredients:

- cauliflower head - 1, florets separated
- olive oil - 1 tablespoon
- Salt and black pepper to taste
- Bacon - ½ cup, cooked and chopped
- tablespoons dill - 2, chopped

Directions:

1. Place the cauliflower in the air fryer; then add the salt and pepper to taste, followed by oil. Ensure to toss well to coat.

2. Cook at a temperature of 400 o F for about 15 minutes.

3. Cut the cauliflower into different plates, then sprinkle the bacon and the dill as toppings.

4. Serve right away.

Nutrition Values:

calories 200, fat 7, fiber 5, carbs 17, protein 7

Hot Butter Broccoli

Preparation Time: 11 minutes

Servings: 4

Ingredients:

- broccoli head - 1, florets separated
- lime juice - 1 tablespoon
- Salt and black pepper to taste
- Butter - 2 tablespoons, melted

Directions:

1. Mix all of the ingredients, gently and thoroughly, in a bowl

2. Place the broccoli mixture in your air fryer and cook at a temperature of 400 o F for a little above 5 minutes.

3. Serve while it is still hot.

Nutrition Values:

calories 151, fat 4, fiber 7, carbs 12, protein 6

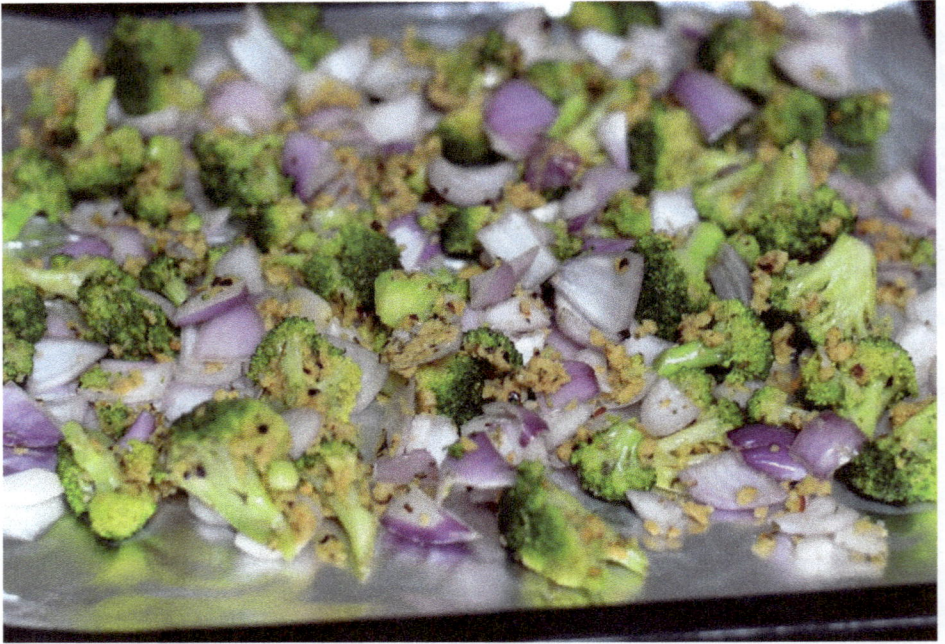

New Potatoes Mix with Toppings

Preparation Time: 20 minutes

Servings: 4

Ingredients:

- new potatoes - 1 pound, halved
- Salt and black pepper to taste
- Butter - 1½ tablespoons, melted
- Dill - 1 tablespoon, chopped

Directions:

1. Place the potatoes in your air fryer's basket, then add the salt and pepper to taste, as well as butter; toss well to coat.

2. Cook at a temperature of 400 o F for 15 minutes.

3. Cut into different plates, then sprinkle the dill as topping and serve.

Nutrition Values:

calories 171, fat 5, fiber 6, carbs 15, protein 8

Seasoned Napa Cabbage Mix

Preparation Time: 17 minutes

Servings: 4

Ingredients:

- napa cabbage - 1, shredded
- yellow onion - 1, chopped
- 2 tablespoons tomato sauce
- Nutmeg - ¼ teaspoon, ground
- Salt and black pepper to taste
- Parsley - 1 tablespoon, chopped

Directions:

1. Put every ingredient in a pan that fits right into your air fryer and mix well.

2. Put the pan in the fryer and cook at a temperature of 300 o F for close to 15 minutes.

3. Divide into different plates and serve right away.

Nutrition Values:

calories 154, fat 4, fiber 4, carbs 12, protein 5

Butter Cabbage

Preparation Time: 17 minutes

Servings: 8

Ingredients:

- green cabbage head - 1, shredded
- butter - ¼ cup, melted
- sweet paprika - 1 tablespoon
- dill - 1 tablespoon, chopped

Directions:

1. Mix every ingredient in a pan that fits right into your air fryer.

2. Put the pan in the fryer and cook at a temperature of 320 o F for 12 minutes.

3. Divide into different plates, serve right away, and enjoy!

Nutrition Values:

calories 181, fat 4, fiber 6, carbs 15, protein 5

Turmeric Kale Recipe

Preparation Time: 17 minutes

Servings: 2

Ingredients:

- Butter - 3 tablespoons, melted
- kale leaves - 2 cups
- Salt and black pepper to taste
- yellow onion - ½ cup, chopped
- turmeric powder - 2 teaspoons

Directions:

1. Put all of the ingredients in a pan that fits right into your air fryer and mix properly.

2. Place the pan in the fryer and cook at a temperature of 250 o F for about 15 minutes.

3. Cut into different plates and serve.

Nutrition Values:

calories 151, fat 4, fiber 5, carbs 15, protein 6

Spicy Cabbage Mix

Preparation Time: 17 minutes

Servings: 4

Ingredients:

- green cabbage head - 1, shredded
- olive oil - 1 tablespoon
- cayenne pepper - 1 teaspoon
- A pinch of salt and black pepper
- sweet paprika - 2 teaspoons

Directions:

1. Place all the ingredients in a pan that fits your fryer, and mix.

2. Put the pan in the fryer and cook at a temperature of 320 o F for about 15 minutes.

3. Cut into different plates and serve immediately.

Nutrition Values:

calories 124, fat 6, fiber 6, carbs 16, protein 7

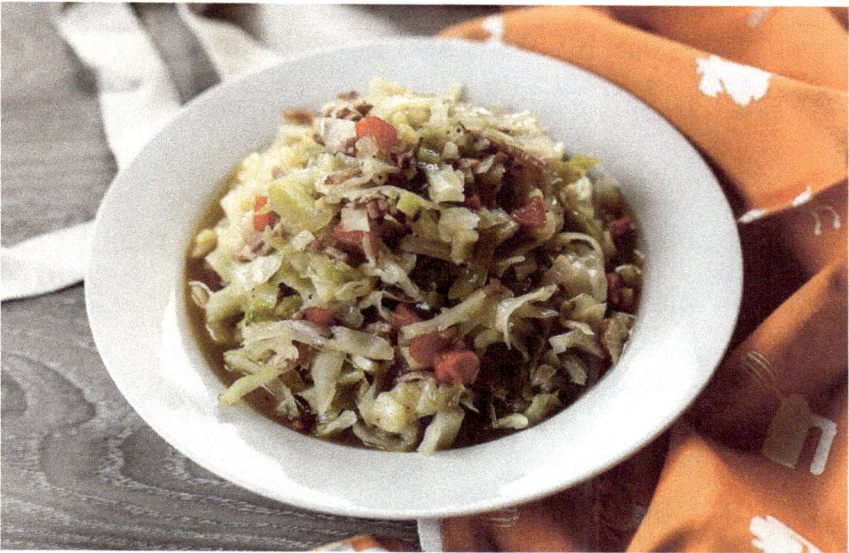

Easy Celery Root Recipe

Preparation Time: 20 minutes

Servings: 4

Ingredients:

- celery root - 2 cups, roughly cubed
- A pinch of salt and black pepper
- Butter - ½ tablespoon, melted

Directions:

1. Place all the ingredients in your air fryer and toss well to coat

2. Cook at a temperature of 350 o F for 15 minutes.

3. Cut into different plates and serve right away.

Nutrition Values:

calories 124, fat 1, fiber 4, carbs 6, protein 6

Seasoned Maple Glazed Corn

Preparation Time: 11 minutes

Servings: 4

Ingredients:

- ears of corn - 4
- maple syrup - 1 tablespoon
- Black pepper to taste
- Butter - 1 tablespoon, melted

Directions:

1. Mix the black pepper, butter, and the maple syrup in a clean bowl.

2. Rub the corn with the mixture, and then place it in your air fryer.

3. Cook at a temperature of 390 o F for a little above 5 minutes.

4. Cut the corn into different plates and serve.

Nutrition Values:

calories 100, fat 2, fiber 3, carbs 8, protein 3

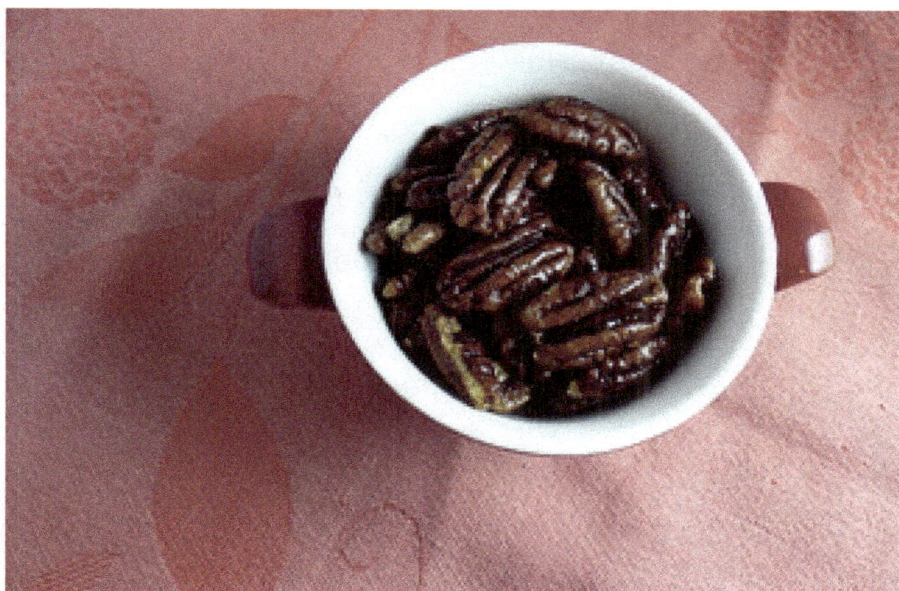

Seasoned Dill Corn

Preparation Time: 11 minutes

Servings: 4

Ingredients:

- ears of corn - 4
- Salt and black pepper to taste
- Butter - 2 tablespoons, melted
- Dill - 2 tablespoon, chopped

Directions:

1. Mix the salt, pepper, and the butter in a bowl.

2. Pour butter mixture on the corn and rub, and then put it in your air fryer.

3. Cook at a temperature of390 o F for a little above 5 minutes.

4. Cut the corn into different plates, sprinkle the dill as topping, and then serve right away.

Nutrition Values:

calories 100, fat 2, fiber 5, carbs 9, protein 6

Seasoned Broccoli Casserole

Preparation Time: 20 minutes

Servings: 4

Ingredients:

- Butter - 2 tablespoons, melted

- broccoli florets - 6 cups

- garlic cloves - 2, minced

- chicken stock - 1 cup

- Salt and black pepper to taste

- fettuccine pasta - 1 pound, cooked

- green onions - 2, chopped

- parmesan cheese - 1 tablespoon, grated

- tomatoes -3, chopped

Directions:

1. Grease a baking dish with butter; the baking dish that fits your air fryer.

2. Add the broccoli, garlic, stock, salt, pepper, pasta, onions, and tomatoes; toss well to coat and ensure to toss gently.

3. Move the dish in the fryer and cook at a temperature of 390 o F for 15 minutes.

4. Sprinkle the parmesan as toppings, divide all into different plates, and serve.

Nutrition Values:

calories 151, fat 6, fiber 5, carbs 12, protein 4

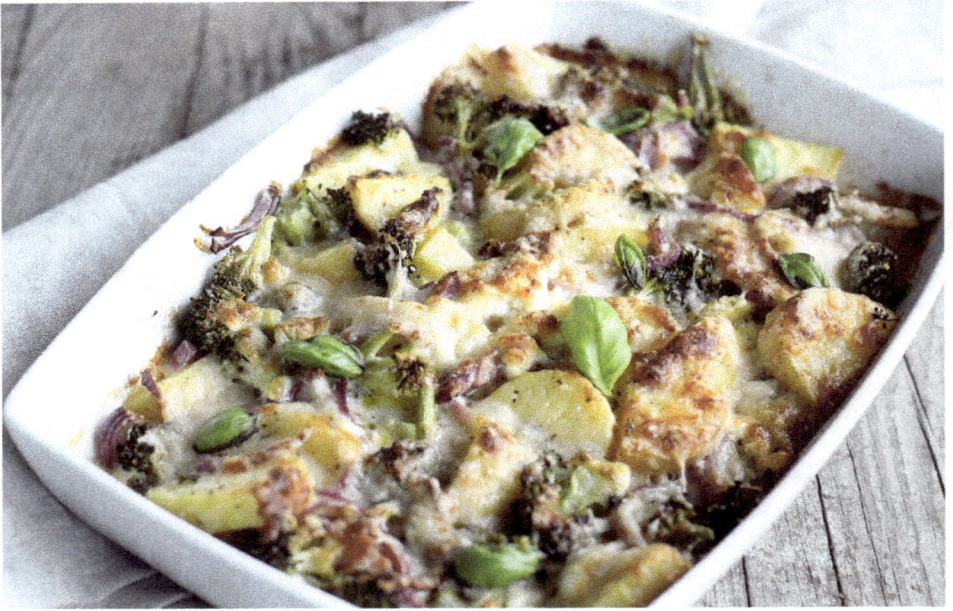

Seasoned Mustard Greens Mix

Preparation Time: 17 minutes

Servings: 6

Ingredients:

- collard greens - 1 pound, trimmed
- bacon - ¼ pound, cooked and chopped
- A drizzle of olive oil
- Salt and black pepper to taste
- veggie stock - ½ cup

Directions:

1. Pour every ingredient to the pan that fits your air fryer and mix well.

2. Move the pan to the fryer and cook at a temperature of 260 o F for about 15 minutes.

3. Divide all of the mix into different plates and serve.

Nutrition Values:

calories 161, fat 4, fiber 5, carbs 14, protein 3

Cherry Tomatoes Skewers Recipe

Preparation Time: 36 Minutes

Servings: 4

Ingredients:

- 3 tbsp. balsamic vinegar
- 3 garlic cloves; minced
- 1 tbsp. thyme; chopped
- 24 cherry tomatoes
- 2 tbsp. olive oil
- Salt and black pepper to the taste
- For the dressing:
- 2 tbsp. balsamic vinegar
- Salt and black pepper to the taste
- 4 tbsp. olive oil

Directions:

1. In a bowl; mix 2 tbsp. oil with 3 tbsp. vinegar, 3 garlic cloves, thyme, salt and black pepper and whisk well.

2. Add tomatoes, toss to coat and leave aside for 30 minutes

3. Arrange 6 tomatoes on one skewer and repeat with the rest of the tomatoes.

4. Introduce them in your air fryer and cook at 360 °F, for 6 minutes

5. In another bowl, mix 2 tbsp. vinegar with salt, pepper and 4 tbsp. oil and whisk well. Arrange tomato skewers on plates and serve with the dressing drizzled on top.

Nutrition Values: Calories: 140; Fat: 1; Fiber: 1; Carbs: 2; Protein: 7

Eggplant and Garlic Sauce Recipe

Preparation Time: 20 Minutes

Servings: 4

Ingredients:

- 2 tbsp. olive oil
- 2 garlic cloves; minced
- 1 tbsp. ginger; grated
- 1 tbsp. soy sauce
- 3 eggplants; halved and sliced
- 1 red chili pepper; chopped.
- 1 green onion stalk; chopped.
- 1 tbsp. balsamic vinegar

Directions:

1. Heat up a pan that fits your air fryer with the oil over medium high heat, add eggplant slices and cook for 2 minutes

2. Add chili pepper, garlic, green onions, ginger, soy sauce and vinegar, introduce in

your air fryer and cook at 320 °F, for 7 minutes. Divide among plates and serve.

Nutrition Values: Calories: 130; Fat: 2; Fiber: 4; Carbs: 7; Protein: 9

Stuffed Baby Peppers Recipe

Preparation Time: 16 Minutes

Servings: 4

Ingredients:

- 12 baby bell peppers; cut into halves lengthwise
- 1 lb. shrimp; cooked, peeled and deveined
- 1/4 tsp. red pepper flakes; crushed
- 6 tbsp. jarred basil pesto
- 1 tbsp. lemon juice
- 1 tbsp. olive oil
- Salt and black pepper to the taste
- A handful parsley; chopped

Directions:

1. In a bowl; mix shrimp with pepper flakes, pesto, salt, black pepper, lemon juice, oil and parsley, whisk very well and stuff bell pepper halves with this mix

2. Place them in your air fryer and cook at 320 °F, for 6 minutes; Arrange peppers on plates and serve.

Nutrition Values: Calories: 130; Fat: 2; Fiber: 1; Carbs: 3; Protein: 15

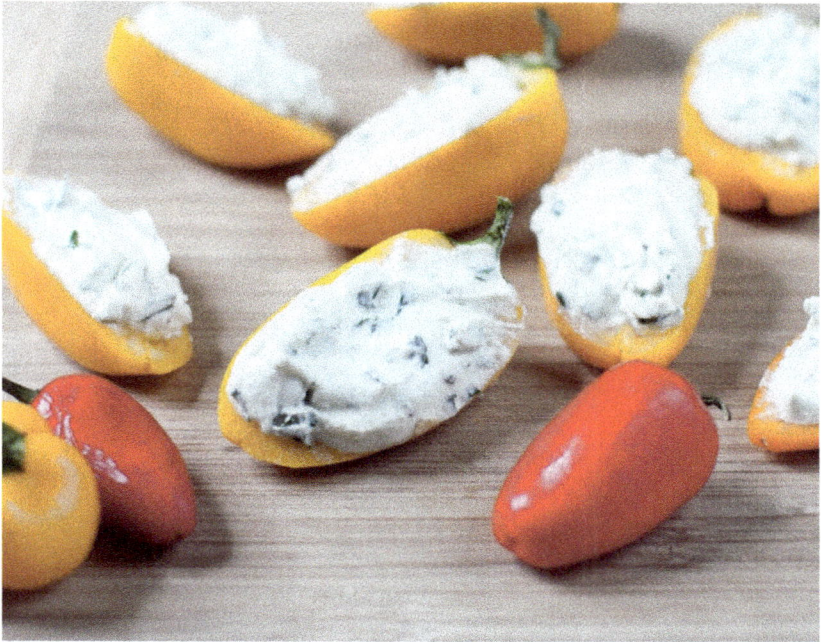

Beet Salad and Parsley Dressing Recipe

Preparation Time: 24 Minutes

Servings: 4

Ingredients:

- 4 beets
- 2 tbsp. balsamic vinegar
- A bunch of parsley; chopped
- 1 tbsp. extra virgin olive oil
- 1 garlic clove; chopped
- 2 tbsp. capers
- Salt and black pepper to the taste

Directions:

1. Put beets in your air fryer and cook them at 360 °F, for 14 minutes.

2. Meanwhile; in a bowl, mix parsley with garlic, salt, pepper, olive oil and capers and stir very well

3. Transfer beets to a cutting board, leave them to cool down, peel them, slice put them in a salad bowl

4. Add vinegar, drizzle the parsley dressing all over and serve.

Nutrition Values: Calories: 70; Fat: 2; Fiber: 1; Carbs: 6; Protein: 4

Herbed Eggplant and Zucchini Mix Recipe

Preparation Time: 18 Minutes

Servings: 4

Ingredients:

- 1 eggplant; roughly cubed
- 3 zucchinis; roughly cubed
- 2 tbsp. lemon juice
- 1 tsp. thyme; dried
- Salt and black pepper to the taste
- 1 tsp. oregano; dried
- 3 tbsp. olive oil

Directions:

1. Put eggplant in a dish that fits your air fryer, add zucchinis, lemon juice, salt, pepper, thyme, oregano and olive oil, toss, introduce in your air fryer and cook at 360 °F, for 8 minutes

2. Divide among plates and serve right away.

Nutrition Values: Calories: 152; Fat: 5; Fiber: 7; Carbs: 19; Protein: 5

Peppers Stuffed with Beef Recipe

Preparation Time: 65 Minutes

Servings: 4

Ingredients:

- 1-pound beef; ground
- 1 tsp. coriander; ground
- 1 onion; chopped
- 3 garlic cloves; minced
- 1/2 tsp. turmeric powder
- 1 tbsp. hot curry powder
- 2 tbsp. olive oil
- 1 tbsp. ginger; grated
- 1/2 tsp. cumin; ground
- Salt and black pepper to the taste
- 1 egg
- 4 bell peppers; cut into halves and seeds removed
- 1/3 cup raisins

- 1/3 cup walnuts; chopped

Directions:

1. Heat up a pan with the oil over medium high heat, add onion; stir and cook for 4 minutes.

2. Add garlic and beef; stir and cook for 10 minutes

3. Add coriander, ginger, cumin, curry powder, salt, pepper, turmeric, walnuts and raisins; stir take off heat and mix with the egg.

4. Stuff pepper halves with this mix, introduce them in your air fryer and cook at 320 °F, for 20 minutes. Divide among plates and serve

Nutrition Values: Calories: 170; Fat: 4; Fiber: 3; Carbs: 7; Protein: 12

Beets and Blue Cheese Salad Recipe

Preparation Time: 24 Minutes

Servings: 6

Ingredients:

- 6 beets; peeled and quartered
- 1/4 cup blue cheese; crumbled
- 1 tbsp. olive oil
- Salt and black pepper to the taste

Directions:

1. Put beets in your air fryer, cook them at 350 °F, for 14 minutes and transfer them to a bowl.

2. Add blue cheese, salt, pepper and oil, toss and serve

Nutrition Values: Calories: 100; Fat: 4; Fiber: 4; Carbs: 10; Protein: 5

Radish Hash Recipe

Preparation Time: 17 Minutes

Servings: 4

Ingredients:

- 1/2 tsp. onion powder

- 1/3 cup parmesan; grated

- 4 eggs

- 1 lb. radishes; sliced

- 1/2 tsp. garlic powder

- Salt and black pepper to the taste

Directions:

1. In a bowl; mix radishes with salt, pepper, onion and garlic powder, eggs and parmesan and stir well

2. Transfer radishes to a pan that fits your air fryer and cook at 350 °F, for 7 minutes

3. Divide hash on plates and serve.

Nutrition Values: Calories: 80; Fat: 5; Fiber: 2; Carbs: 5; Protein: 7

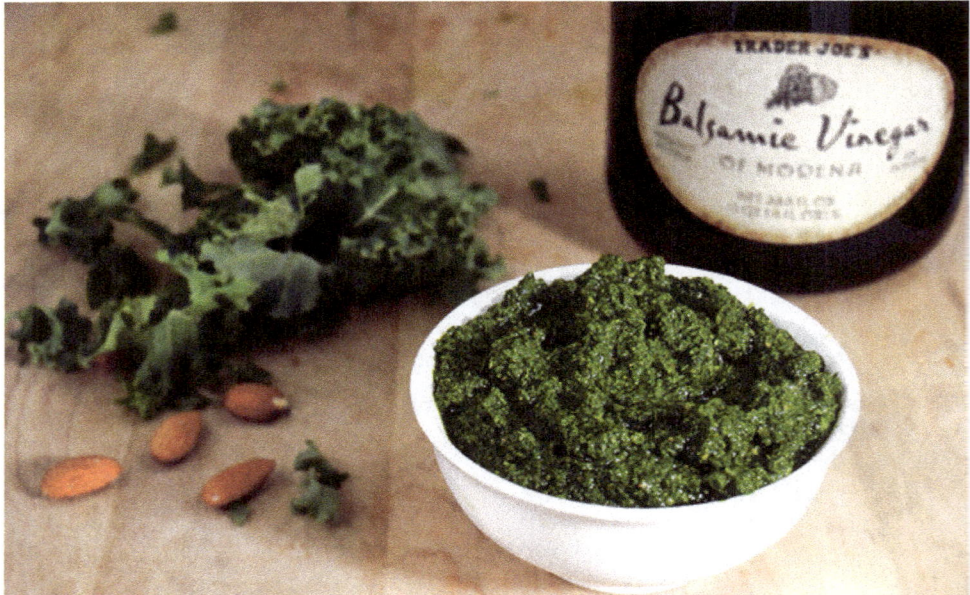

Flavored Fried Tomatoes Recipe

Preparation Time: 25 Minutes

Servings: 8

Ingredients:

- 1 jalapeno pepper; chopped
- 4 garlic cloves; minced
- 1/2 tsp. oregano; dried
- 1/4 cup basil; chopped.
- 2 lbs. cherry tomatoes; halved
- Salt and black pepper to the taste
- 1/4 cup olive oil
- 1/2 cup parmesan; grated

Directions:

1. In a bowl; mix tomatoes with garlic, jalapeno, season with salt, pepper and oregano and drizzle the oil, toss to coat, introduce in your air fryer and cook at 380 °F, for 15 minutes

2. Transfer tomatoes to a bowl, add basil and parmesan, toss and serve.

Nutrition Values: Calories: 140; Fat: 2; Fiber: 2; Carbs: 6; Protein: 8

Mexican Peppers Recipe

Preparation Time: 35 Minutes

Servings: 4

Ingredients:

- 4 bell peppers; tops cut off and seeds removed
- 1/2 cup tomato juice
- 1/4 cup yellow onion; chopped
- 1/4 cup green peppers; chopped.
- 2 cups tomato sauce
- 2 tbsp. jarred jalapenos; chopped.
- 4 chicken breasts
- 1 cup tomatoes; chopped
- Salt and black pepper to the taste
- 2 tsp. onion powder
- 1/2 tsp. red pepper; crushed
- 1 tsp. chili powder
- 1/2 tsp. garlic powder
- 1 tsp. cumin; ground

Directions:

1. In a pan that fits your air fryer, mix chicken breasts with tomato juice, jalapenos, tomatoes, onion, green peppers, salt, pepper, onion powder, red pepper, chili powder, garlic powder, oregano and cumin; stir well, introduce in your air fryer and cook at 350 °F, for 15 minutes

2. Shred meat using 2 forks; stir, stuff bell peppers with this mix, place them in your air fryer and cook at 320 °F, for 10 minutes more. Divide stuffed peppers on plates and serve

Nutrition Values: Calories: 180; Fat: 4; Fiber: 3; Carbs: 7; Protein: 14

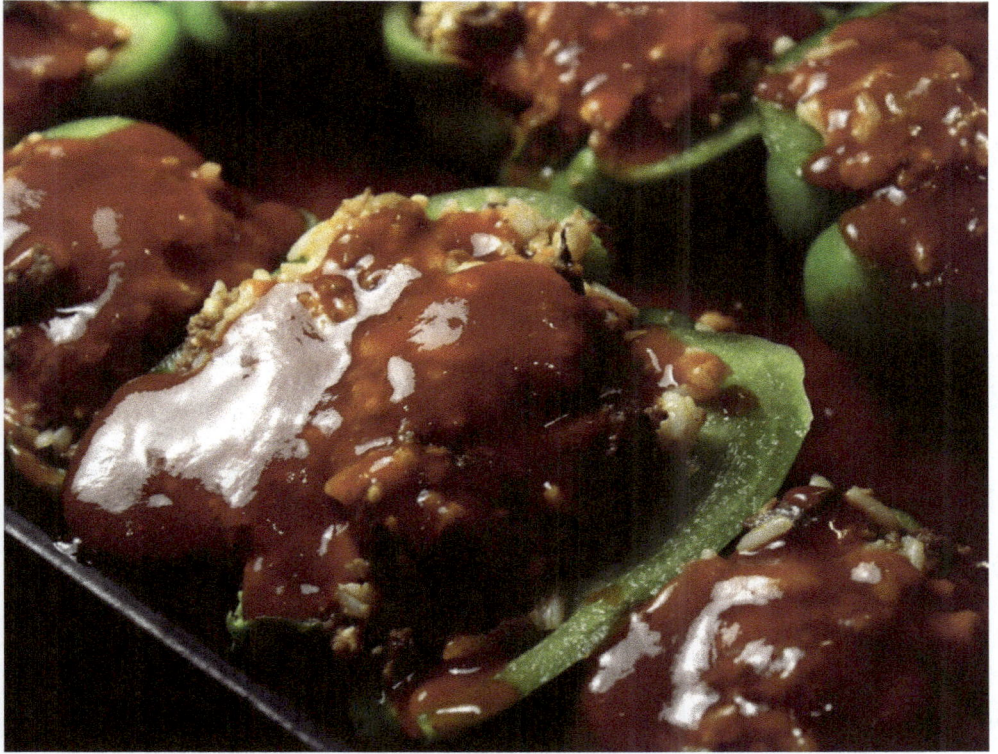